ADORABLE FAT GIRL SHARES HER WEIGHT LOSS TIPS

Bernice Bloom

Contents

Dear readers,

Hello, my name's Bernice Bloom. It's presently quarter past six on a soft summer's evening and I'm lying on the floor doing leg lifts while I catch up with Made In Chelsea. And if that little nugget of information hasn't left you reeling in your seat then you don't know me very well. Me – exercising in my own home? Squeezing in a little bit of gentle exercise while I relax over skinny, posh people in the evening? Incorporating exercise into my everyday life...exactly like they tell you to in every article about fitness ever written. Me – doing something right? Yes – I know – I don't understand what's happened to me either.

But – somehow – despite years of failing to lose more than three pounds before instantly putting eight pounds back on again, I have got myself sorted and I've managed to properly lose weight. I feel amazing...not thin – not by a long way, I've lost half the weight I need to lose so there's still a way to go, but I've lost a lot, and losing weight is definitely an incentive to lose more weight because every pound you lose gives you confidence that you can lose more, so I'm full of hope that I'll lose the rest of it and soon be deliciously slim and probably giving Kate Moss a run for her money.

If you've read the novels about my character Mary Brown's exploits, you'll know that she joined a Fat Club and it transformed her life. Not only did she meet a whole load of thoroughly lovely people who she went on a lot of crazy adventures with, she also bagged herself a delicious new boyfriend (he's gorgeous!) and - crucially - she managed to shift the piles of lard that had settled on her stomach, thighs and hips. She did it by following the five steps that they taught her at Fat Club and I'm going to explain them to you now. Everyone at Fat Club lost weight and you can too.

This book also contains advice and stories from readers who have contacted me, and a Q&A of the five most frequently asked questions I get, and what my answers are...

I hope you enjoy the book, and find it useful

Bernie x

INTRODUCTION FROM MARY BROWN, STAR OF THE ADORABLE FAT GIRL SERIES:

Before I lost weight, I used to wonder how people did it. I mean *really* wonder... I would see someone in the paper who'd lost two stone, or bump into an old friend who I hadn't seen for ages, and discover they had lost weight, toned up and were looking fantastic. And I'd think – how have you done it? HOW ON GOD'S FREAKING EARTH HAVE YOU DONE IT?

And the fascinating thing is, when I thought 'how have you done it?' I didn't mean it literally because I knew exactly what they'd done – they'd eaten less and exercised more. We all know what to do to lose weight.

You know how the body works and I know how the body works. I know that if you put in less than you take out, you'll lose the weight. Simple! But – no, no, no – because the maddening truth is that it's very hard to do...not simple at all.

So when I saw someone who had lost weight, what I asked myself was – how did you mentally convince yourself to do what millions of us want to do?

What I wanted from them was a tip, a clue, as to how they did it. I was dying for one magical little secret that would help me. I really didn't need them to say 'Eat broccoli, not a chocolate bar.' I didn't need to hear that they got off the bus a few stops early and walked up the stairs.'

I KNOW ALL THAT. TELL ME WHERE THE MAGIC KEY IS THAT WILL UNLOCK, IN MYSELF, THE ABILITY NOT TO EAT ALL THE TIME.

In the search for the magic key I went to Overeaters Anonymous and there I discovered the five tips for losing weight that have transformed my life. I'm going to tell you right off the bat what they are, then in this little book, I'll go through them in much more detail, and explain what it all means, with examples of how the people I met on Fat Club and various readers who have written in to me, got them to work. Then all you have to do is follow them and lose tonnes of weight, then next time your friend sees you she'll scream HOW HAVE YOU DONE IT? And you'll be able to smile and say 'yeah...it's all because of Bernice Bloom and Mary Brown,' and I'll be famous and be invited to garden parties at Buckingham Palace. Everyone's a winner.

OK. So, the five tips are:

- Understand what your body wants
- Psych yourself in instead of psyching yourself out
- Be nice to yourself; treat yourself with respect
- WAW! Water and walking
- Making it a habit

Nice and straightforward? Not yet, but it will be. I promise, promise, promise it will be.

One of the things that going to Fat Club gave me was a confidence in my ability to lose weight. When everyone is positive around you, it's amazing how that rubs off and you feel positive too. I stopped beating myself up and started accepting that I wasn't overweight because I was greedy, lazy, slovenly or useless. I was overweight because I used food to make myself feel better, feel less bored, less lonely or less vulnerable.

The key thing that I did when I realised that was to break the emotional connection between food and feeling good. I started thinking of food as being exactly what it really was, instead of what it represented to me. Then I could start transforming myself into the person I wanted to be. Food is just there to stop you being hungry; that's all. Keep saying that to yourself...that's all it is. FOOD IS JUST TO STOP HUNGER. Say it, say it again. SHOUT IT.

You can lose weight if you only use food to combat hunger. Deep down you know you can do it. Face it, you can do anything if you really want to.

I mean, people have done extraordinary things in the world. People do crazily complicated wild and wonderful things every day. I've seen the news – blokes air ballooning round the world, swimming the channel and women giving birth to quadruplets on top of a mountain and things like that. Running marathons? How do people do that? I'm the same species as all these people yet I can't run further than the kitchen without needing open heart surgery and a lung transplant. I knew there had to be a way of me harnessing the power that other people seem to have naturally, to make myself focus on a weight loss campaign. There had to be a way I could do it.

I knew that I really must be able to change my outlook on the world, and get out of the bad habits I'd got into...stop eating the leftovers purely out of habit. Stop clearing everything on my plate because that's what I'd always been told to do as a child. I wasn't a child - I was a 20-stone woman. I had to learn a new approach to food.

What I learned more than anything from Fat Club was that people become overweight for lots of different reasons - eating too much ice cream, drinking too much, wolfing down too much chocolate...but the thing people have in common is that they are overweight because food has become more than nutrition to them.

If that's you, please read on...perhaps you've eaten when you're lonely, or bored, or you eat because the children are playing you up, eat because your boss is a pain. You might be eating to fill a little hole inside you that sits there because you don't feel loved or happy or worthy. You know that food doesn't help you but you eat it anyway because it's a quick and easy way to feel instantly full, protected and satisfied.

This is not a diet book – heavens, there are a million diet books out there – the world doesn't need any more. This is a book that should motivate you, comfort you and help you.

I happen to think it's a very important book because it will make you feel much, much better about yourself while you're losing weight and I happen to think that feeling good about yourself is the most important thing in the world, and certainly the thing that will help with weight loss..

Food is many people's way of reaching out, psychologically, for something to make them feel warm and happy and loved. Tell me – how the hell is a diet book that tells you to eat spinach leaves instead of chips going to help you feel warm and loved? It's not about understanding what to eat, it's about how to feel nice without reaching for cake. It's about breaking the habit.

If you are overweight it's not because you're a bad person, you didn't kill anyone, you didn't steal anything, or hit anyone, or do anything criminal. You just ate too much because you felt low, or got into a habit of eating while bored. That's not a crime. Most importantly, it can be changed. Reading this book is a great start because it will show you examples of lots and lots of people from my Fat Club and from readers who changed, and explain how they did it.

I really hope it helps you, I know it will make you feel better about yourself, and make you realise that 90% of the battle is about loving yourself a bit more and not feeling the need to medicate with food, silence the pain with food, or kill time with food. And it's simpler than you think...lots of people have written in to me and told me that they did it, and their stories are in this book, and I did it too!

This book is divided into five sections based on the five tips outlined earlier. At the beginning of each section is an explanation of the way in which that tip helped me, then stories from other people who have written in to me to explain how they lost weight.

MOST FREQUENTLY ASKED QUESTIONS

Before we get going on the details of what you need to do to lose weight, I thought it would be useful to run through some of the questions I am most frequently asked when people hear that I have lost so much weight. I'm assuming that some of these questions will be on your mind:

Q: *How do you stop yourself bingeing? When I go off the rails and eat a McDonalds or a pile of chocolate, I end up eating loads, absolutely tonnes. I can't help myself. I'm OK when I don't eat those foods at all, but when I start eating them it's all over and I just can't stop.*

A: Yes, I'm with you. We're all the same to greater or lesser extent. There are several reasons for this. First, it's important to realise that most of the time you're not eating because you're hungry but for emotional reasons – because you're sad, lonely, heart-broken, miserable or plain bored. Food WILL NOT HELP with these emotions, so you end up eating loads in a quest to dampen the feelings. Trying to separate out hunger from emotional eating is an important part of cracking the weight loss issue.

The other thing is that even if you are eating because you are hungry, heavily processed food full of trans-fats, colourants, sugar and artificial foodstuffs won't give you the right nutrition so you will stay hungry. We'll go into all this much more later in the book, but when you get hungry your body is after nutrients. If you give it nutrients, the hunger pains will drift away. But, if you don't give yourself the proper nutrients, you'll continue to feel like you need to eat, even though you've already eaten tonnes and tonnes.

You can eat cheese burger after cheeseburger in McDonalds and feel like you want to eat more and more because your body is still craving nutrients. It's had lots of food, but not lots of nutrition.

The other problem with highly-processed food is that it is digested very easily without the body having to do any work. Normally, when the body is digesting natural foods, it sends a signal to the brain to say when it's full, but if food is very processed and the body doesn't have to do any work, the food is eaten before the stomach lets the brain know that the body has the food it requires, so you can eat way more before you feel remotely full.

So, the answer, I'm afraid, is to eat the best, healthiest food you can. If you feel you want to eat loads – allow yourself to do that, but only binge on healthy stuff – eat carrots, humous, avocado – really tasty food stuffs, but stuff that is good for you. You simply won't be able to eat as much of it as you can McDonalds and will feel full surprisingly quickly (I know what you're thinking – the idea of carrots and hummus v McDonalds is a no-brainer, but give it a go. Don't count calories, don't try to control yourself, just eat the best, most healthy food you can find, and eat until you're full and don't want to eat any more).

Q: I feel exhausted when I diet and exercise, so I end up having to take time out at work to cope. What can I do?

A: Taking time out is not such a bad thing! It's particularly not a bad thing if you're exercising and trying to live a healthier life. I try to take time for myself every day. I call this *Bula Time*. This is not some bizarre Buddhist theory or weird tribal thing, it comes from a place called Turtle Island in Fiji (can there be a more alluring name for a place?)

This beautiful slice of Pacific Ocean paradise sits indulgently, bathed in glorious sunshine, in the Central Yasawas area of Fiji. Like so many of the country's islands, it has breathtaking, long, white, sandy beaches fringed by azure water and an income derived from coconut farming. But there is something that distinguishes this island from the rest of Fiji – it is an hour ahead. It has been operating on its own unique time system since Blue Lagoon was filmed there in 1980, and everyone involved in the shooting had to get up an hour earlier to catch the sunrise. Such is the way with these small Fijian Islands, that no one really thought it worth bothering to change things back once the filming was over, so Turtle Island has kept Blue Lagoon time ever since, and the villagers still get up sixty minutes before the rest of Fiji. They call it 'Bula Time' – meaning time for 'health', 'life' and 'vibrancy'. They use the extra hour to focus on themselves, relaxing and being good to themselves. I suggest you do too!

Q: I hate myself so much when I mess up on a diet. I'll eat one bite of chocolate then fall into a cycle of self-hatred that is beyond my understanding, and the only way I can fight my way out of it is to eat and eat and eat until I quieten the angry voices by weighing them down with food

A: This, in my opinion, is the reason that most diets fail...because people aren't kind enough to themselves and they don't allow themselves to make even the slightest mistake.

Most diets don't fail because we all lack willpower, or are greedy, or have fat genes, they fail because the psychological spin that we are thrown into when we stray from the path, defeats everything. In every day life we mess up all the time, but as soon as we mess up, even slightly, on our diets – that's it – whole packets of biscuits are devoured, bottles of wine are opened and take-aways are called.

The truth is, if you're eating healthily and exercising whenever you can, the occasional bite of chocolate isn't going to be a problem. It's what you do 80% of the time that will define what size you are.

So, if you slip up, smile it off. It doesn't matter. Be nicer to yourself. Don't think that because you've made a mistake it makes you unable to lose weight.

Those who succeed in sport always say that the most important the lesson they learned, and the one which made them successful, was that just because they failed at something, it didn't make them a failure.

This is an important concept to grasp.

If every time a footballer missed a goal, or a cricketer missed a catch, he thought "that's it, I'm useless, I'll never make it, I'm going home" he'd never be able to play, let alone reach a high standard.

It's really important to remember, when you're trying to get fit and healthy and lose weight, that you can't be perfect all the time. You'll miss the goal occasionally, there'll be a hand ball or two along the wall. You won't hit every ball for six. SO WHAT? No one is perfect. You will have times when it doesn't go so well – just shrug them off. Enjoy the chocolate while you're eating it and try to get back to being as healthy as possible the next day. Don't beat yourself up about eating. EVER. In fact, don't beat yourself up about anything. EVER.

Stop those horrible voices in your head saying you can't do it, smile, laugh it off, put on some lipstick and get back to the healthy eating the next day.

SECTION ONE: UNDERSTAND WHAT YOUR BODY NEEDS

OK, this is where the fun starts...your first step to a whole new body. I want to begin by telling you about my trip to a safari last year. (see <u>Adorable Fat Girl on Safari</u>)

When I was out in the wilds, watching the animals, the thing that struck me most of all was how none of them were fat. NONE of them. Not one single animal. If you sit in any cafe in town and people watch, you'll see all range of sizes pass by; certainly you won't have to sit there for very long before seeing someone who is overweight Why is that? What are animals doing that we are not?

Happily, on safari, there was a rather handsome ranger on hand to explain:

The main reason that animals aren't overweight is because they don't eat more than they need. They eat to live. If an animal has just made a kill, he eats that animal, then doesn't go out to make another kill until he's hungry again. The relationship between animals and food is that they eat because food is the fuel to keep them going. They don't eat because the alpha lion has gone off with a young female, because they're bored or because they feel depressed. They eat when they are hungry.

How do they know when they are hungry? The same way as we do: hunger pains. Hunger pains are your best friend! Learn to love them and cherish them.

Those pains or rumbles we feel are designed to tell us that some time soon it would be good to have some food. They are a sign that you are ready to eat. Honestly – I know this sounds ridiculous – but those rumbles and pains are really important.

Conditioning has taught us that when our stomachs rumble it's a bad thing, and that we shouldn't let ourselves get so hungry that they rumble. Yes we should! The truth is that those hunger pains are a good thing. They indicate that your stomach wants food soon. They are a warning that you're getting low on fuel (it's like the fuel gauge on the car moving down – you're not about to stop through lack of petrol, but it would be good to put some petrol in the car in the not-too-distant future).

Treating food as fuel and eating when you feel hungry are the keys to survival in the wild. Could they be the key to weight loss too?

Over the next couple of weeks, try only to eat when you're hungry and at least once a week, make sure your stomach rumbles before you eat. Just try it. Give yourself a loud cheer every time you hear your stomach rumble...it's a good thing – welcome it and celebrate it.

The third point I want to make in this section contains what you should eat. What is your body asking for when you feel hungry and get those hunger pains? Fuel. Exactly like when a car asks for fuel. You can't just shove crisps, pizza and chocolate into a car engine or you'll run into problems, and you can't just shove crisps, chocolate and pizza into your mouth either, without there being problems.

Try hard to remember this: when you feel hunger pains your body wants nutrients. If you eat a big fruit salad or plate of vegetables,, you may not feel the same satisfaction as if you eat great big bag of chips, but you will give your body the nutrients it wants so you won't get as hungry later. You could eat a whole loaf of bread and it would fill you up, but your body won't feel satisfied because it won't have had the nutrients that it needs, so the hungry feelings will emanate again, as your body asks for nutrients again. If you eat rubbish again, the body will say it's hungry again an hour later, as it realises it doesn't have the nutrients it needs in the food you've supplied. So, you'll eat more and more and get fatter and fatter and always be hungry. Does that sound like you? It sounds a lot like I used to be. And it's a horrible way to live; always stuffing yourself full of food, and always feeling hungry and unsatisfied. Stop it now!

YOUR BODY ISN'T BEGGING FOR FOOD – IT'S BEGGING FOR NUTRIENTS, SO THAT'S WHAT YOU NEED TO GIVE IT.

So – just to summarise – three things to remember:

- Think of the safari animals and try to think of food as fuel. Just eat to fuel yourself when you get hungry and pick the best fuel.
- Try to wait for hunger pains or at least murmurings of hunger before you eat. Treat hunger pains as real triumphs.
- Remember what the pains mean – they mean that your body needs nutrients...not just any old food – you won't be satisfied if you eat any old food, eat the most natural, unprocessed, healthy food you can, then the hunger pains will dissipate, the weight will fall off, you'll feel better and healthier and won't be drawn to unhealthy eating in the future.

I found the key to losing weight was to think about what my body needed, not what my mind or my emotions required. My body needed nutrients so that's what I gave it. As much food as I wanted, as long as everything I ate was doing me some good.

Here are some stories that readers have shared about their weight loss journeys and their keys to success with food control. I hope you enjoy their stories...

Sarah's story:

Hi, my name is Sarah. I'm 52-years-old and I have lost 54lbs. I went from 196lbs to 142lbs. I did it by not being a dustbin!

I'd tried to lose weight loads of times before, but would lose some weight, then get fed up, stop, and put it all back on again. Then, I did it. I lost the weight and kept it off because of one simple saying that has really worked for me - don't be a dustbin. It's quite simple, but that's the rule I have...and it's worked. I write DBAD on my hand every morning, and am conscious of it all the time. I urge you to try it – just implant that saying into your mind.

My story:

I realised I had a problem around food when someone saw me finishing the leftovers from a Chinese takeaway we'd had, and said "how can you still be hungry?"

The question took me by surprise - of course I wasn't hungry - we just had a huge meal, but I carried on eating just because it was there. I'd got it into my head that it was better if I ate the leftovers than threw them away. A mixture of not wanting to waste food that was there, and habit. It seemed daft to leave a couple of spring rolls and some spoonfuls of seaweed behind – so I just put them into my mouth despite not being at all hungry.

My friend said "the leftovers belong in the dustbin", and it suddenly struck me that I was treating myself a bit like a dustbin. Why was I shoving bits of food I didn't want into my mouth? Habit.

If there were any bits of bread lying around, or if there was a piece of pizza left -- I would eat it. I wasn't hungry, lonely, sad or any of the other things that drive you to eat. It was just habit that I'd shove any leftovers into my mouth. The kids would leave their crusts – I'd eat them. I'd serve up dinner and there'd be a little left in the pot – I'd eat it. Gradually, I'd put on a hell of a lot of weight.

So, I decided to stop. I created my DBAD label and set about trying hard to break the habits of a lifetime. It was much easier than I thought it would be. I think what happens when you start thinking to yourself "I will not be a dustbin" is it you think more carefully about everything you're putting into your mouth. Will this do me any good, or am I eating it because it's there? Why am I eating it? It forces you to take that two minute break before shoving something into your mouth that forces you to think about whether you really need it or want it.

Try it. As you're making dinner, don't shove bits of food into your mouth while you're cooking – have more respect for yourself. You're not a dustbin.

I've found that my habit of just eating any leftovers or anything left on the side disappeared when I refused to treat myself like a dustbin anymore. It also made me think about the whole concept of having "leftovers", and food lying around that could easily tempt me. I've got three teenage children, so I do a big supermarket shop every week, but what I've tried to do is be really specific about what to buy in the weekly shop -- what do I plan to cook for the meals that week? What do I need to buy?

Rather than wandering around and grabbing things off the shelves and throwing them into my basket, I think about the meals we are going to eat. I think DBAD as I'm walking down the aisles. Shopping properly means eating properly - it means there's less food being wasted, and less chance of me hoovering it up.

This in itself has definitely made a difference to the amount I'm eating, but I think it's more the fact that I am a subconsciously thinking before I eat that is making a real difference.

The gradual process of making yourself look at food differently means thinking about what's best for you. I started to think of fruit and veg as being treats, because they make me feel better and look great and so are the opposite of being a dustbin. Shoving bits of old pizza left in the box into my mouth, and the remains of a Chinese takeaway was never going to make me feel better – that stuff belongs in the bin, not in me.

If you shove pieces of cake in your mouth to make you feel better for five minutes, the impact of it can be colossal -- you stop caring, you don't value yourself. You start using food to make yourself feel better. I'd never have been able to do it by thinking about it logically – I did it by having a strict rule – don't be a dustbin, and the rest came naturally.

Just think about it... of all the things in the world you might want to be -- why would anyone want to be a dustbin? Everytime you feel yourself behaving in a dustbin like fashion -- stop it. Become aware of any dustbin like tendencies.

There is no one reading this book who wants to be a dustbin, so stop it!

As I said, I wrote DBAD on my hand to remind myself "don't be a dustbin" -- it started to apply to everything I put into my mouth. Was I eating this because it was good for me, or was I just being a dustbin? I found this tactic really worked. This is a simple thing, but sometimes it's the simple things that people say that click something in your mind and make you behave differently.

The other thing about this small saying is that it's not setting you off on a tightly calorie controlled diet, or making you run six miles a day. It's just subtly getting you to alter your behavior around food. If someone has got a handful of chips left on their plates - don't eat them, you are not a dustbin. You are worth more than that. Much more than that.

Pippa's story: Four golden rules

Hi, my name is Pippa. I'm 58-years-old and I have lost 43lbs. I went from 183lbs to 140lbs. I did it by being incredibly strict with myself and following these four golden rules.

My story:

I'm not the sort of person who normally follows rules; if I'm making a cake, I find it really hard to follow the recipe, I like to throw things in a mixer and see what it tastes like. But somehow, perhaps because my mind is so chaotic and in need of order, I found that when I set myself very clear rules to follow, I was able to lose weight. I call these my four golden rules, and I took to wearing four gold-coloured bangles to remind myself constantly of these four rules. I think that if you are going to follow strict rules, you need to remember them all the time, and it was a constant reminder to me, every time I reached out to food, and saw the four bangles jangling on my wrist.

So, my four rules... these are my tips to you; if you follow them you will lose weight. Let me repeat that: YOU WILL LOSE WEIGHT. Now if you decide not to follow them, or that all sounds like too much like hard work, that's your decision but I'm telling you that these rules work. As I've already said, if you're the sort of person who thinks they might forget, a good way is with the four bracelet or four bangles approach.

My first golden rule was - when I was hungry I allowed myself to eat. But I could only eat when I was hungry; I didn't allow myself to eat until I was hungry. This helped teach me when I should be eating. If other people were eating and I wasn't hungry, I'd stop myself. I'd looked down at my bangles, and remind myself that I could only eat when I was hungry ... when I could feel that hunger building up in my stomach.

The second rule, which goes hand in hand with this rule, was that I had to stop eating when I wasn't hungry anymore. I ignored all the rules from childhood, that you have to finish everything on your plate, and just ate until I wasn't hungry anymore. Remember, if you get hungry again, you can have more food. There's no shortage of food. This took a bit of getting used to, and I realised that most of the time when I'd eaten less than half of the food on my plate I wasn't hungry anymore, I was fine, but I was eating it because it was there. If you can stop yourself (look at the bangles) make yourself put your knife and fork down when you are no longer hungry, you'll find it makes a huge difference to the amount you consume. I think, looking back, that most of the food I was eating wasn't because I was hungry, but because it was there.

So, they are the two main golden rules. If you can follow them, you'll lose weight.

The other two rules I had were in order to make those to work.

So, rule number three was that I should eat whatever my body felt it needed. I was sure that my body would direct me to what it needed if I stopped just guzzling whatever was in front of me. I'd realised this when I was pregnant with my first child, and got mad urges for certain sorts of food as my body tried to feed the two of us. If the body was capable of doing that when I was pregnant, then clearly it was capable of doing it once I'd had the baby. I might just have to listen a bit more carefully for the cues. Now, if I am really hungry, and really fancy carbohydrates, I won't stop myself. If I'm hungry, I eat, but I try to eat what I feel my body wants me to eat, and – ofcourse – I stop when I'm full.

My final rule, the final gold bangle on my wrist, is probably the nicest, but it's also very important - that rule is that I should really enjoy the food I was eating. So if I had a plate of food, I should relish all the different tastes and really enjoy it while I was eating it, rather than shovelling it down and feeling guilty about it as I had before. But then stop when I wasn't hungry anymore.

I made myself eat properly at a table and not while distracted at my desk, on the train, or while walking down the street. If you eat while you're reading a book or flicking through a newspaper, you're distracted from the process of eating, and you never know when you're full. Jangle those bangles, lay out a proper table, sit down and enjoy your food, but make sure you only eat when you're feeling hungry, and always stop when you're not feeling hungry anymore. I promise you – that's all you need to do.

Susan's story: I found my inner caveman

Hi, my name is Susan. I'm 22-years-old and I have lost 32lbs. I went from 164lbs to 132lbs. I did it by finding my inner caveman!

My story:

Yep, I was really put off by the name – why can't it be called Cave woman diet? I really don't want to look like a caveman, but I do like the idea of going back to nature and trying to eat as healthily as possible, but not if it involves a big beard, a hairy chest, and clubbing wild animals to death before I can eat.

My doctor mentioned the diet to me, and I shrugged and smiled in the surgery and said "yes, of course I'll try it", but obviously had no intention of doing anything of the sort. I needed to lose weight because my blood pressure was high (and my weight was too high ... and it had become increasingly clear that there was a link between the two highs!).

The doctor was talking about getting me onto pills to control my blood pressure. I said I didn't want to do this – I had a friend who'd taken blood pressure pills and ended up with terrible depression. I wanted to avoid that. So I knew I had to lose weight. He suggested the caveman diet, so I left the surgery, went home and researched it on the computer.

The thing that struck me about all the descriptions of the caveman diet was that it was a real commonsense diet... a healthy approach to trying to lose weight. It seemed to have a very straight forward, logical backbone to it and easy rules to follow.

Nothing to do with calories or pilates classes. You didn't have to sit there and wonder whether you could eat egg yolks on a Wednesday, protein on a Friday or drink alcohol after 11pm ...just eat as if you were a caveman!

For those of you who are wondering...this means eating natural, unprocessed foods – meat, fish, eggs, berries, nuts, veg – these are the foods that our body was designed to eat, and anything else we put inside ourselves makes us fat. At least that's the message I told myself to keep things simple. And it worked. I had a hellish first week, yearning for bread, cakes and pasta, but then that passed and I started to feel better about myself and much fuller than I had before.

Then, a really interesting thing happened; I had to go to a friend's wedding and I had a huge blow-out - I drank all day on an empty stomach, picking at high fat canapés, crisps and dips, and then having the biggest meal in the evening with tons of pudding and loads of cake, I drank way into the evening then we went for fish and chips on the way home. I felt like I was treating myself ... letting myself go from this diet I'd put myself on ... but, honestly, the next day I felt so bad it made me realise just how great I'd been feeling on the caveman diet.

It took me a couple of days before I felt myself again, and I haven't wanted to go out on a limb since. The weight has fallen off me. I feel happier, healthier, my senses are more alert ... I just feel brilliant. When I went back to the doctors, my blood pressure had dropped right down so I didn't need to take the blood pressure pills.

The thing that appealed to me about the diet was that it is not in the least complicated ... if you keep in your mind just to eat what a caveman would have eaten, that's all you have to do. So, you are in a restaurant and you are given the choice between fish and vegetables, and pasta carbonara ... you know which one the caveman would have been able to have - so have that (fish and vegetables!).

As well as being called the caveman diet, I've also seen this referred to as the clean diet. You are eating clean food (in other words -- foods that have not been processed or messed with). Cavemen wouldn't have been able to make coffee cake, donuts or Mississippi mud pie. But they would have been able to get hold of plenty of berries and nuts.

You might be reading this and thinking how dull this all sounds. I promise you it's far duller to be 30lbs overweight, and facing all the potential health hazard as well as high blood pressure. And it's easy - you have to just remember one thing - would a caveman have been able to eat this?

When cavemen ate it was to feed their bodies to keep themselves alive, and keep themselves as healthy as possible. That's not a bad premise for any diet.

Martin's story: Strict calorie control, but eating whatever I want

Hi, my name is Martin. I'm 30-years-old and I have lost 42lbs. I went from 246lbs to 204lbs. I did it by counting calories. It doesn't sound like much of a tip, but I think it's the easiest way to do it. Just be strict with yourself – give yourself a calorie target every day, and take it one day at a time. Don't worry about the long haul or what about Christmas, what about the summer holidays – just focus on the here and now, and making sure that every day you don't go over your calorie ceiling. If you do that, you will lose weight.

My story:

I know people say that calories aren't equal – there are good calories and bad calories – you are supposed to avoid calories with fat and sugar in and eat calories with vitamins and protein. I know that, I really do, but it's very complicated trying to work out what you can and can't eat, and worrying what to order in a restaurant and turning into a madly fussy eater who only eats spinach. I found it much easier to set myself a daily calorie limit and stick to it.

I allowed myself 1500 calories a day, and that was it. I had 300 calories for breakfast (scrambled egg on toast, usually), 500 for lunch and 500 for dinner, and 200 for a drink or a snack. I just did that every day and I lost weight.

My gut feeling is that people complicate it too much. It all gets horribly difficult when you're told that avocados are fattening...but they're good for you. Nuts are full of goodness, but fattening. It's hellish to work out what you can and can't eat. I found it easier and straight forward to play the numbers game.

Let's face it, you can get fat from eating healthy food too. Count the calories – just do it, stick to it and the weight goes – problem solved.

Mandy B's story: Love your kitchen

Hi, my name is Mandy. I'm 60-years-old and I have lost 40lbs. I went from 190lbs to 150lbs. I did it by revisiting my whole approach to food, and cooking much more at home, so I knew exactly what was going into it, and by enjoying new flavors. So, basically, my tip is – learn to love your kitchen!

My story:

I lost weight properly when I fell in love with cooking, and being in my kitchen. It was only when I really started to get to grips with cooking for myself, and making tasty food that was low in fat and low calorie, that I managed to shift the weight.

I think there were two psychological bonuses to preparing things for myself ... first of all, putting effort into cooking things properly for myself made me feel special when I was eating, and not as if I was denying myself tasty foods constantly. The second bonus came because I just became more aware, generally, of food and tastes. I found that my taste in food changed and I wanted to eat healthier foods, foods that were better for me.

These were the key things I did –

1.   I grew a herb garden. I know that sounds a bit dull, but if I was only eating salads, it was nice to have them with tons of coriander on them or home-grown mint and parsley. The mint was lovely for fresh mint tea. I grew chilis that were great for spicing up vegetable stew

or rubbing onto chicken before grilling it to give it a bit of a tang.

2.   I bought lemon and lime. I cut right down on the fruit I was eating because I was eating tons of it, and obviously it's full of sugar. I know it's good for you, but I was eating way too much. Lemons and limes had all the goodness without the sugar. I'd squeeze lemon into hot water to drink in the morning and use lemons and limes to flavour foods ... either by squeezing them, or grating the zest into dishes. I promise you it makes a real difference when you start cooking nice food for yourself, instead of buying diet versions of normal food. It's hard to feel looked after and cherished when you're buying frozen diet food. If you're chopping coriander, rubbing chilli on to chickens and squeezing lemons and limes into food it makes it all much more exciting and palatable.

3.   I bought mustard and horseradish and, like I said earlier, grew my own chillies. The reason for these spicy foods is that they help any food that might otherwise be bland. When I grilled a whole load of vegetables, I would put a half teaspoon of horseradish into a cup with a few dessert spoons of boiling water mix it all up and pour it over the vegetables while they were grilling then I'd serve them on a bed of coriander and mint with a squeeze of lemon and it tasted absolutely gorgeous... full

of taste (which I think also helps you feel full up which is why I would avoid all dull diet foods if I were you!!!)

4.   I controlled the portions I was having. If I was eating things that may lead to me putting on weight, like pasta or potatoes, I was able to weigh them out or measure them out. The key to getting the right portion, is to have a portion the size of your fist, no bigger. When you go out to eat they will give you way too much food and it's very hard not to eat it. Also, once you learn the whole concept of portion control no food is really off limits.

5.   If you have a chicken breast, but don't want to eat all of it, slice it long ways rather than in half. I know this sounds daft - you are getting the same amount of food, but if you cut a chicken breast in half it looks like half. If you slice it down the middle it doesn't look as if you are cheating yourself out of half a breast of chicken. The same goes for a baguette... instead of having a short stumpy piece of bread have a longer piece but only half of it, then you feel as if you've had a proper meal.

6.   I tried to buy vegetables that I have never tried before ... and seek out the freshest food around. I now go to a market on Saturday afternoons to buy loads of lovely fresh vegetables, in season, that hasn't been flown halfway around the world. I bought a coconut last night and had a go at cooking chicken and Coconut milk with chilli. By the time I added garlic, onion, broccoli and

spinach, I had a huge bowl of comfort food that was really delicious with coriander sprinkled on the top. Honestly -- I promise you -- it's the way forward if you want to lose weight.

7.   I bought spicy pepper blends which I sprinkled onto popcorn and other low calorie treats. The taste is there without the calories. It worked for me!

SECTION TWO: Psych yourself in instead of psyching yourself out

This second section looks at the psychological issues involved in weight loss...how do you convince yourself not to eat what you really want to? How do you stop yourself from reaching for the crisps, cake, takeaways and bread basket, when every fibre of your being urges you to do so?

For me, the way I coped, and broke the link between emotional well-being and eating was by repeating phrases to myself, like 'I only eat when I'm hungry', 'food is just to stop hunger' over and over and over until my emotions caught up with my voice. It will happen, and it will lead you to questioning what you're doing. If you bite into a big cream cake when you're not remotely hungry, while chanting 'I only eat when I'm hungry, a part of you will start to feel uncomfortable. You'll find yourself questioning what you're doing, and once you start questioning, the logical side of you will take over from the emotional side, and you'll find it easier to talk yourself out of eating all the time.

So, whenever you're confronted by food that you fancy eating, try to slip into the habit of chanting 'I only eat when I'm hungry, I only eat when I'm hungry.'

Even if you eat the big cream cake, try to keep chanting while you're eating it and you will feel a disconnect and that will help you to stop yourself next time. But you need to do the chanting. If you do it frequently it WILL work.

Certainly that was my experience. Getting a psychological advantage over eating too much was a real help to me. It was the experience of these people, too:

Claire's story: I did a psychological make-over

Hi, my name is Claire. I'm 42-years-old and I have lost 38bs. I went from 178lbs to 140lbs and I did it by sorting my head out! In short, I gave myself a psychological make-over. My tip to you is to do the same – you need to sort your head out if you're to have any chance of getting rid of that tummy!

My story:

My tip to you is to think very carefully about why it is that you have got fat. I know that sounds like a silly question – it might well be because you've eaten too much! But considering all the dangers of being overweight, why have you allowed this to happen? You might be shrugging at this point and thinking you'll skip over this section but please don't. Because I found that once I'd worked out what psychological problems I had that were leading me to eat too much, I was in a much better shape to sort out issues surrounding the amount I ate and drank.

I hope that doesn't sound too heavy, but I also used to be hopeless with money, socialise too much, and eat and drink way too much. When I stopped and did what I call a "psychological makeover" (PMO) I found myself much more in control ... not just with money and going out socialising all the time, but also with eating and drinking. I'd just lost control of my life, in so many ways, and desperately needed to get it back.

My psychological makeover came from spending time with a friend who had been an alcoholic, and had been in treatment, and knew what it took to get him off alcohol. He talked to me about the way in which his life was examined and analysed by those treating him, and the changes it led him to make. I took on board everything he told me about the course, and I worked out whether there were any lessons that I could learn from them. The answer was a very resounding – yes!

These are the things I did as part of my eight stage PMO:

dreams
mask
negativity
selfishness
stress
settling
waiting
laziness

Write them down, one below the other, with room to write alongside them, and jot notes about your own life as I explain. I promise this will help you.

Dreams - I wasn't being true to what my own dreams were. I'd always wanted to work in fashion, but I knew my parents would frown, so I had taken a job in a post office, then moved to a bank. I had a decent job, with a decent income, good work hours and friendly coworkers, but I wasn't living the dream I'd always had for myself. I knew I had to change this and live my life for me.

Mask – this ties into the first point really, but I discovered that I was showing the world what I thought they wanted to see – a professional, sensible, sophisticated woman with a good job in the bank. That wasn't me. I was effectively wearing a mask and being what I thought people wanted me to be rather than who I was.

Negativity – there's no doubt that there were a lot of negative people in my life, people who made me feel worse about myself when I spent time with them. I knew I had to cut them out.

Selfishness – I was living a selfish life, a life just for me. I changed things, and weaved in some charity work that made me feel much better about myself. Feeling more positive about myself, and confident in myself, was a key to making me want to treat myself better, and eat more healthily.

Stress – there's no doubt that I was really sweating the small stuff. Worrying about whether I'd put the bins out in the right place, had I told the milkman I wanted skimmed milk, did I remember to do things on time... stressing things that really didn't need to be stressed about. I knew I needed to relax, take a deep breath and learn to let go of things which really didn't matter that much.

Settling - is there anyone who hasn't done this one? I knew I was settling for a job I didn't like, in a relationship that had nothing to inspire me, and a life that didn't really fulfil me. I decided to try not to settle ... even if it meant being on my own, that was better than settling for someone who I wasn't madly in love with.

Waiting -- I was very good at this! I kept saying I'd go onto a fashion design course, or start making my own clothes, or save up for a sewing machine, or go to the gym ... tomorrow. I spent a lot of time waiting for tomorrow that never came. I've learnt that if something is worth doing is worth doing now. Just start, don't spend your life forever waiting.

Laziness - I realised that instead of feeling sorry for myself for being in a job I wasn't wildly keen on, I needed to get out there and change things. Things weren't going to change by themselves ... whether that be my weight, my job, my life or my prospects. Don't be wishy-washy, vague and lazy. If you want it: go out and get it. If you change your life for the better, you'll find that everything will fall into place, and the need to eat will disappear and your motivation to get slim and healthy will appear.

Mike's story: The three-week watershed

Hi, my name is Michael. I'm 38-years-old and I have lost 50lbs. I went from 252lbs to 202lbs. I did it by eating smaller meals. I'd tried to lose weight loads of times before, and this time I was successful because I gave myself three weeks to get started. My tip is – if you can get yourself across the three week barrier, you can do it. Bear than in mind when you're on a diet, fed up and wanting to stop...keep going for three weeks!

My story:

I tried to lose weight ... cutting out the pints of beer, the takeaways and the fried breakfasts, thinking about everything I ate, and trying to cut down to smaller, healthier meals. I was doing well for a week, then weighed myself and discovered I'd lost one pound. One pound!

It felt like a kick in the teeth. I'd dramatically altered the way I eat and all that happened was that I lost one pound. If things kept going on like this I wouldn't lose the weight I wanted to lose until I was about 120-years-old.

Needless to say, like 1 million people before me, I gave up, went back to the pub and back to my old ways. I enjoyed the takeaways and a few pints with my mates and decided I must be one of those people who just can't lose weight.

The way I broke the cycle of dieting for a short period of time, getting fed up, stopping, then doing the whole thing again, was when someone said to me that you have to give yourself time to get started. You have to do whatever you're going to do to lose weight for three weeks minimum before you come to a judgement on how it's going. Whatever you decide to do ... whether it's

Weight Watchers, the Cambridge diet, healthy eating, cutting back carbs, whatever it is - do it for three weeks before forming a view. You have to. The simple fact is - if you can't guarantee to do it for three weeks, you will not survive, because those first three weeks are crucial.

It takes a little while for the impact of what you are doing to register on the scales. It might register straightaway, like my one pound loss, or two pound loss, but that isn't enough incentive to keep going. I managed to crack it by not weighing myself for three weeks then when I got on the scales after three weeks I'd lost 7lbs. That was massively motivating, made me want to carry on, and reaffirmed that I was doing the right thing. The weight loss didn't carry on at that level, I had some good weeks and bad weeks, but I was able to endure it because I got those three weeks in at first so that my routine of weighing myself every Monday started with me already having lost seven pounds, so already feeling motivated.

I urge you to give yourself time. Don't do what I kept doing, and dieting for seven days expecting to see tremendous results, getting pissed off when there are no real changes, and falling back into old eating habits. It's taken quite a long time for you to put your weight on ... certainly with me it crept slowly over about three years

- is it too much to expect that you give it three weeks of dieting to begin the process of getting rid of it?

So, just to repeat my psychological tip - decide what you're going to do – as I've said, I did it by cutting out all the things I knew were bad for me and having smaller meals - then give yourself three weeks before you judge it.

It's just three weeks ... you can do it.

Stick to it for three weeks then weigh yourself or measure yourself and come to a view. I think that 99% of people will have lost some weight after three weeks – enough weight for them to feel happy with the way the first three weeks have gone and inspire them to carry on.

The same theory applies when you're a few months into the diet, and you have a bad gym day, or a bad eating day, or you end up in the pub with your mates can't resist that fourth pint of beer... it took you years to put this weight on, one bad day isn't going to derail it. Shrug it off and get back on the bandwagon. No matter how badly you slip up, it doesn't matter, you've only lost control when you decide to lose control. You have it within you just shrug it off and carry on again.

Maria's story: I worked out the difference between emotional eating and eating for hunger.

Hi, my name is Maria. I'm 26-years-old and I have lost 34lbs. I went from 164lbs to 130lbs and I did it by realizing that I wasn't eating because I was hungry, but for emotional reasons. I identified when those times were, and I stopped doing it.

Note from Bernie: there were so many responses from people saying that the way they lost weight was to get control of their emotional eating that I have included two tips on coping with emotional eating. This is the first one ...

My story:

I was well aware that I was eating for emotional reasons, and not just because I was hungry. I was comfort eating. I'd reach out for food when things weren't right – when I was stressed, lonely or sad. The food made me feel immediately better, but, over the years, it had led to me putting on a lot of weight, which had the effect of making me feel more stressed, sadder and lonelier! I knew this in my head, but that didn't seem to make any difference to how I behaved...as soon as I was stressed, I ate. Worse than this, eating so much made me feel bad, so I'd eat more to overcome the bad feelings, and end up feeling even worse.

So, I was in the classic cycle of overeating. The trouble was that this was something I'd always done. I didn't think I'd ever be able to work out the difference between feeling hungry and wanting to eat, and feeling lonely, sad or fed up and wanting to eat. How would you ever know the difference? If there was food around, I wanted it. I knew that if my stomach rumbled I was hungry, but I wasn't aware of any other subtle signs about whether I was hungry or just eating for emotional reasons.

It was when I managed to distinguish between my emotional eating and my eating because I was hungry, that I made the breakthrough, and lost the weight. So my tip to any would-be dieters is: work out when you're eating for emotional reasons and when you are eating because you're hungry. Once you can do that, it's much easier to stop doing it.

So – how do you do it? This is what I did:

First of all, I wrote down everything I ate and how I was feeling when I ate. It started off simply - I had a bagel for breakfast, a cheese salad roll for lunch, then a packet of crisps Twix and more sandwiches at 4pm.

Why did I suddenly eat so much?

When I looked at what was happening, I realised that 4pm was the time that my husband phoned me and told me that he couldn't get back in time to pick our kids up from school. They have clubs til 5pm, so I would have to leave at 4:30pm to pick them up, meaning leaving work early. My instant response was to eat. Instead of saying to my husband "no, you promised you do it, you have to pick the children up," I rushed out and ate loads.

I was worried about letting my boss down by leaving early, worried about the kids, and annoyed at my husband. Without stopping to think, I filled the emotion and upset with food.

Most worryingly of all, as I kept the diary for a few weeks, I realised that eating was my primary emotional coping mechanism. If I became upset, lonely or bored, I'd eat. I'd eat when I felt stressed, carry on eating when I was full, and start eating whether I was hungry or not. Basically I was eating to feel better.

I felt hopelessly out of control around food, and once I started eating to fill emotional voids, I couldn't stop. I'd want to eat and eat and eat until I felt better. It was almost as if I was loading the food on top of the problems to stop them bothering me. I was creating a layer that separated me from the world. I loved the feeling that stuffing myself gave me, but I hated the feeling afterwards - the resentment, self-hatred, and anger at my lack of control. I had to learn to identify when I felt this emotional hunger, before I could begin to try not to eat.

It took quite a long time for me to work it all out, but these are the things I discovered along the way about the difference between emotional hunger and physical hunger.

* First of all, physical hunger arrives gradually. You feel a little bit hungry, then a little bit more hungry until you are really quite peckish. Emotional hunger hits you like a thunderbolt; one minute you're fine, you get a negative phone call or have a negative thought and - boom - you've eaten three packets of chips before you can work out why you've done it.

* When it comes to emotional hunger, you'll be driven to eat a certain type of food. I went carbohydrate crazy... not sweet things, but big jacket potatoes stuffed with loads of cheese and coleslaw, pizza, chips, takeaways ... if you are truly physically hungry, you are not anywhere near as particular about the sort of food you want - an apple, a piece of bread - they are all fine. Emotional hunger demands a particular sort of comfort food.

* Emotional hunger is out of control ... you can't say to yourself that you'll have a couple of chips - the whole lot has gone. I found that I didn't even really enjoy the taste of the food, I hadn't really noticed I was eating it, I was just shoving it inside myself to make myself feel better.

* The key thing that I've found with emotional hunger vs physical hunger was that emotional hunger was never satisfied ... I'd keep eating and eating and eating way beyond feeling comfortable and I'd want to keep eating as much as I could.

* Emotional hunger isn't located in the stomach. Rather than a growling belly or a pang in your stomach, you feel your hunger as a craving you can't get out of your head.

* Emotional hunger often leads to regret, guilt, or shame. When you eat to satisfy physical hunger, you're unlikely to feel guilty or ashamed because you're simply giving your body what it needs. If you feel guilty after you eat, it's likely because you know deep down that you're not eating for nutritional reasons.

So my tip is to identify all the times you eat for emotional reasons. Use a food diary, and think about all the points I've listed above. After that, you need to work out how to stop your emotional eating. I admit that I did it by joining the lighter life program – a very low calorie weight loss program which a lot of people don't agree with. I found it was useful for me to take all the food out of my diet so I wasn't around food, couldn't think about food, and dismissed it from my life. Simultaneously, the lighter life people talk to you about how to gain control around food. The whole thing really worked for me, and I feel much happier now, but when I look back at the craziness I used to have when I was around food it's almost like someone on drugs looking for their next fix – it meant everything to me to get the sort of food I wanted and to eat it quickly until I was so full I was almost sick. Obviously, if you feel like I did, you might want to see your GP or a psychiatrist to talk through the issues. But the first thing to do is just to be clear and honest with yourself about whether you are eating for emotional reasons rather than physical. Good luck.

(the second emotional eating story)

Patricia's story: I stopped my emotional eating

Hi, my name is Pat. I'm 46-years-old and I have lost 48lbs. I went from 208lbs to 160lbs and I did it by realizing that I wasn't eating because I was hungry, but for emotional reasons. The big thing I did which allowed me to lose weight, was to stop my emotional eating. Now, I know that doesn't sound like much of a tip ... of course we all know we could lose weight if we stopped our emotional eating, but what I did that I'd like to pass on to you as my number one tip, is that I identified exactly how, why, and when I fell into patterns of emotional eating. Once I'd done that, getting some sort of control over my food intake was quite straightforward. And after that, losing weight was much easier.

I suppose I knew I was an emotional eater because I was eating way too much, way beyond the point of satisfying hunger, stuffing myself with food for the sake of it. But I didn't realise that it was called "emotional hunger" and I just thought I was insanely greedy, and couldn't work out why. I'd be getting on with my life, then somehow I'd be overwhelmed by this need to eat, or a thought would enter my mind and that was it ... I couldn't relax until I'd eaten something, and not just something, loads and loads of food until I felt so completely full up I couldn't move - really fattening food - all the sorts of foods that anyone with a weight problem would work really hard to stay away from. I felt completely out of control around these foods, and compelled beyond all common sense to eat and eat and eat. I simply had to eat.

I didn't feel able to do anything about the fact that I ate until I could understand why I did it. I didn't know why this was happening. Like I say, I thought of myself as being greedy which just made me feel worse than ever. Then, I realised that what I was doing was emotional eating, and worked out a way to stop it.

My story:

I began by going to see my GP, because I went to join the gym and discovered by their measuring and weighing techniques that I was "morbidly obese". I was definitely obese, but didn't really think of myself as being really huge, and I think part of me always thought that I could do something about this if I really tried.

Hence my attempts to join a gym. The people in the gym were lovely, but said they would feel much happier if I went to see my GP first, just to check that he was happy for me to start an exercise program. When I went to see my GP and started talking to him, he asked me what sort of food I ate in the day, and I replied, quite honestly, that in a normal day I might have fruit and cereal for breakfast, a sandwich or jacket potato for lunch, and then usually a salad or jacket potato in the evening. He looked at me above his half moon glasses and raised his eyebrows.

"Can I be honest with you?" he asked me.

"Of course," I replied.

"You wouldn't be this size if you ate like that," he said.

That's when I explained to him that the food intake I had described was a normal day, but that there were lots and lots of very abnormal days when I went absolutely ballistic around food. He leaned over and touched my arm, and said "why do you think you eat like this?" that's when I burst into tears, and said I didn't know.

I have no idea why I burst into tears, and I was madly embarrassed at having done so, but looking back at that moment now, four years on, and having lost over 45lbs, it was the best moment of my life. He got me to explain to him how disciplined I could be with food, but then sometimes, for no reason at all, I'd go absolutely mad and need to eat gross amounts of fatty food. He said he thought this was emotional eating, and whilst it would be useful for me to start on a diet and exercise program, I also needed to take a good look at the emotions that were causing me to eat. He recommended a psychologist.

I'm crying as I'm writing this, because the truth is that the psychologist he sent me to see changed my whole life. If you think you may have the same issues that I have, I'd recommend going to talk to your GP. He can put you in touch with a psychologist on the NHS... in the meantime, read on, and I'll tell you how it all worked for me.

I turned up at the psychologist's office feeling a bit of an idiot ... I didn't know what she was going to ask me, or what I was going to say. I didn't have any big worries or issues. My parents haven't split up, I haven't lost my job, I didn't have any real money worries. I was just this fat girl who couldn't stop eating.

She made it very clear that she thought there were underlying issues related to my need to eat in such large quantities. We talked about the whole thing, and in my instance she became very clear that it was my inability to have proper relationships with men that caused a great void in my life which I was filling with food. We did a lot of talking about past relationships, and things that had gone very wrong in them, and I continue to see her to talk about all these issues. But she was very keen to help me as quickly as possible with the over-eating, so she helped me to try and work out what the triggers were for me to overeat.

She explained that most emotional eating is linked to unpleasant feelings, but it can also be through positive emotions. Some people eat too much when they're feeling very happy, because they feel relaxed and happy and want to continue the happiness, and reward themselves for the lovely feelings they have.

It soon became clear that this wasn't what I was doing. It was unpleasant feelings that made me eat too much. After much talking, thinking, and analysing, it became clear that I was feeling sadness, anxiety and loneliness, and that was what was forcing me to eat.

She said that I was numbing myself with food ... avoiding emotions I'd rather not feel. This might not be what you are doing ... other people eat when they are stressed. Apparently there is a biological reason for this – cortisol is the stress hormone released when you feel worried or under pressure, and this triggers cravings for foods which give you a burst of energy. If you feel like stress in your life is completely out of control, you may feel that the eating you do to compensate is equally out of control. I want to emphasise that I'm not a psychologist -- I'm just telling you my story about what I learnt when I tried to take control of my over-eating. The other thing that can cause emotional eating is boredom or feelings of emptiness ... filling a void in your life. It occupies you, and distracts you from any dissatisfaction you may be feeling.

There are other, bigger issues, of course. People can start overeating when a parent dies, or they go through a traumatic experience. In my view the only way you are going to work out what it is that forces you to overeat is to keep the most detailed emotional eating diary you possibly can or to talk to a psychologist. You need to try and work out what the patterns are behind your emotional eating. They might be really subtle.

One thing that provoked a turnaround in my understanding of my eating was when I had a complete binge after chatting to a friend on the phone, and she said she had to go. I felt immediate emptiness and loneliness (except that I didn't, of course, because I stuffed these emotions down by eating everything I could find in the fridge). It's not always big dramatic events that throw you off course, but little things, like when you're chatting to a friend, and she has to go. Her saying she was going seemed like a rejection and it triggered this descent into mad eating.

I kept details of how I felt, what I wanted to eat and what I actually ate.

I found I would stuff myself with food when I went to family functions, or when I was facing a big night out with more glamorous friends. On many occasions, I got off the train to go to a social function, headed straight into a kebab shop, bought myself tons of food, and then just got the train back home without going to the function. Why was I doing that? What was I scared of? It seemed to all come back to worrying about relationships with men.

It helped me enormously simply being able to identify these emotions. Then I had to try and kick the habit of going from that emotion to eating. I did that surprisingly simply. The psychologist said that a lot of people have a lot of problems breaking the link, but I found that by doing things like putting my feet flat on the floor and breathing deeply for a minute, or getting on the phone to another friend, helped enormously.

For me, the tip that led to my massive weight loss was finding out what it was that made me overeat. The rest seem to take care of itself. If you find yourself in the position I was in, or if any of this resonates with you, I wish you lots and lots of luck. You can make yourself feel much better, lose the weight, and start to have a happier life. Go down to your GPs and see whether anyone there can help you. Lots of luck and lots of love.

Charlie's story: Get a reality check

Hi, my name is Charlie. I'm 28-years-old and I have lost 56lbs. I went from 182lbs to 126lbs and I did it by grabbing my life by the horns and sorting myself out. Brutal, but effective!!

My story:

My tip for losing weight is quite brutal -- I know this will sound very hard and difficult, but it is: get a reality check. That's my tip to you – get a reality check.

I was very overweight (I'm only 4'10"), but kind of lying to myself about just how big I was. I avoided mirrors, kept away from people taking photographs, and never got on the scales. It allowed me to think that actually things weren't too bad, but the truth is that if you are avoiding looking in full-length mirrors, and diving out the way anytime anyone pulls a camera out, you might not be dealing with reality!

My reality check moment came at a wedding ... no place for escape. When I was told that I had been picked to be a bridesmaid, my first thought was "no no no no no" there's absolutely no way I can walk down the aisle in a dress with everyone looking at me. But then another part of me reassured me that I could easily lose weight in time for the wedding, and actually it might be quite a good thing to have a function that I really wanted to lose weight for ... it might give me the motivation I need to lose weight.

So, I accepted the kind invitation, and put off the first bridesmaid fitting thinking that if I could delay it a bit, I could lose weight. It didn't happen. So in the end I had to go along and have the bridesmaid dress fitting. I shut my eyes and put my hand over my ears as they did the measuring, and refused to look directly into the mirror. This continued throughout the process of preparing for the wedding, but on the wedding day I put my bridesmaid dress on, not having lost any weight at all, and walked down the aisle after my friend – a little ball waddling along behind her.

That was all fine ... no mirrors in church, no need for me to face how big I had got. But then came the real horror, and the moment when I got the biggest reality check of all - the photos came back from the wedding. I was huge. I mean it. I was literally twice the width of one of the other bridesmaids. I really was enormous. It was the reality check I needed, because even though I'd been aware that I was overweight, I hadn't taken it really seriously. As I looked at myself I realised that this wasn't just about losing a couple of pounds to fit into a smaller bridesmaid's dress, I had a real problem. I had to get myself back into shape because the size I was in those pictures was very unhealthy.

That shocking moment forced me to take weight loss much more seriously than I had done ever before. I weighed myself and discovered that I was 182lbs (I was convinced that I was around 150lbs), then I took a good look at myself in the mirror, and looked at the clothes I was wearing - all of them baggy, designed not for their beauty or flattering nature, but to cover me up. How had I let this happen?

The truth is that I had let this happen by ignoring the facts. I wasn't dealing with reality. My tip to you is to look in the mirror and get on the scales, get yourself a measured, and deal with the truth of the size that you are. Don't lie to yourself. It's much harder to commit yourself to lose weight and to do all you can to get fit and healthy, if you're refusing to acknowledge how overweight you are in the first place. I'm sorry if this all sounds brutal, but I do think a lot of us choose to ignore the signs, and make life doubly hard for ourselves by avoiding reality.

In the end, after my shock reality check, I managed to lose the weight by making small changes. I cut out sugar to start with.... I let myself eat what I wanted, but only things without sugar. The next thing I did was cut out white foods -- particularly pasta, bread, biscuits and potatoes. By this time I was starting to lose weight, so felt motivated to stick to it. Then someone mentioned to me that alcohol has a lot of sugar in it, so I decided to try and cut right down on that. Instead of having wine, I had vodka and tonic, first of all because wine comes in a bottle, and once I've got it open I can't stop, and also because vodka and tonic has less sugar in it.

I kept doing that – cutting back on the bad things gradually, until I was eating a really healthy diet, then I introduced exercise, and the weight just drifted away. I had a few plateaus, of course, and I managed to fight through those, and I had a lot of moments where I almost slipped, and moments when I actually slipped – having fish and chips and half a bottle of wine, but I managed to get back onto the diet again the next day. I never kidded myself that I was only losing a couple of pounds – I knew I had a lot of weight to lose, and I knew it was important that I lost it. It was this honesty with myself and facing up to the reality that enabled me to finally lose the weight for good.

SECTION THREE:

Be nice to yourself; treat yourself with respect

I think this is a much misunderstood area of weight loss. People who are overweight beat themselves up every day, they feel bad about themselves and wish they didn't look the way they do. Overeating and lack of control around food are desperately difficult to deal with because food is available around us all the time...we can't get away from it. I don't wish to belittle those who have drug or alcohol problems, but dealing with those issues means abstaining from them...food is very different. You have to eat; there is no choice. That means that you have to operate around food all the time, deciding what to eat. If you make bad decisions, you beat yourself up, but unlike an alcoholic who might fall off the wagon every few months, you have the propensity to fall off it every five minutes because food is in and around us all the time. It means you're beating yourself up and feeling awful all the time. By beating yourself up all the time, and feeling bad about yourself and a failure, you will end up eating more to make yourself feel better and to push down the negative feelings about yourself. So you get caught in a vicious circle. You can start to break this by being kinder to yourself...don't beat yourself up!

You might also have a negative self-image because of the way that overeating has made you look. Overeating shows itself so clearly. You look fat and feel uncomfortable so you feel furious with yourself. Your way to cope with feeling furious is to eat, makes you feel worse and more and more fed up.

Well - don't worry. Relax. The world hasn't ended. If you're jeans are tight it's not the end of the world. Just stop, breathe and don't call yourself horrible names.

You've got this. Here are some techniques for feeling better when the world around you feels pretty horrible.

Sonia's story: Meditation

Hi, my name is Sonia. I'm 39-years-old and I have lost 32lbs. I went from 170lbs to 138lbs. I did it by going to Weight Watchers. I found it quite stressful keeping an eye on everything I was eating and counting up the points, and kept getting fed up, stressed out and giving up. Then, I'd find some motivation from somewhere and start again, but the same thing would happen – I'd get fed up with it, miss a few weeks, and stop. In the end I managed to stick to it for one reason, and I'll share that with you now. I've lost most of the weight (I've got around 7lbs to go). And the thing I did? I started meditating.

My story:

I was about 40lbs overweight and fed up with life. I couldn't think of a way of losing weight, because every time I tried, I gave up. Nothing seemed to motivate me. I found I'd had the best luck with Weight Watchers, so I decided to try that again. I began well, as I always do, but then started to get fed up, stopped doing it for a few days, and never got back on it. I just didn't feel I had control over my food intake...eventually the food would win!

I'd be great for a couple of weeks then would wreck all my days of good dieting by suddenly eating a load of food, or drinking a load of alcohol, even if I wasn't hungry, and that was it – diet over, all ruined.

I remember one time when I'd been really good for couple of weeks, eating healthily, and going for regular walks, and cutting out the pub visits, then I had a really tough day at work, ran to catch the train home and just missed it. The next one wasn't for 40 minutes, and before I'd even thought it through, I was in the fish and chip shop eating a huge bag of chips and curry sauce while I was waiting. Once I was three quarters of the way through it, I decided I wanted more, so went to the newsagents and bought a chocolate bar, then went to the pub and had two large glasses of wine. I then got on the train, feeling really sick, and just desperately confused about what it was made me do that. I wasn't hungry. I wasn't planning to eat, but it was as if one little knock-back had ruined everything. If the train had come into the platform, I'd have just got on it, but the disappointment and annoyance of missing the train just made me lash out and reach for food and drink.

And it wasn't as if I could stop myself – it was almost as if I had the food and had eaten it before I realised what I was doing. I seemed to be suddenly in the fish and chip shop and then halfway through a large packet of chips before I had even thought about whether I was hungry. The more I thought about it, I realised that incidents like this were quite common – I was out of control.

Realising this came at the same time as I saw a leaflet about mindfulness and meditation, and it had the simple message "get control of your life again". It struck me that that was exactly what I needed to do ... so I went along and learned to meditate.

Anyone who's not tried it, I would strongly advise it ... either download a YouTube video, get a book, or if you see classes on, go along and try it out.

It's not weird and wacky men in orange suits wailing and chanting – it's just a bunch of stressed out people who feel their lives are running away from them and want to get control.

The main thing that meditating did for me was to teach me to stop and think before doing things. It's given me the ability to pause for just a second, which makes all the difference. I can close my eyes and clear my mind of all the mad thoughts, breathe, and be more logical, less emotional.

I'm more relaxed and happier. I feel more in control and I've stopped using food as an emotional crutch. It takes a bit of practice, but I started by doing it in bed for five minutes at nights, and in the morning for five minutes before I get up. It helps me to clear my mind.

I seem to have more clarity and an emotional balance which, certainly for me, has helped me to be much more sensible about healthy food choices, and has led to me losing all the weight I wanted to.

Anyway – that's my tip. And my big, big message to you is to give it a go. We all know that answer to weight loss is in the mind, so why not just spend 10 minutes a day decluttering the mind and helping yourself enormously to live a healthy, happy life. Good luck!

Anna's story: Get positive

Hi, my name is Anna. I'm 48-years-old and I have lost 50lbs. I went from 225lbs to 175lbs. I did it by getting positive and starting to like myself. Sounds a bit wishy-washy but I worked out that I was over-eating to make myself a happy person. I made the conscious decision to be a happy person, and losing weight was easier. Sounds odd? Read on...it's free and it worked for me!

My story:

One of the things that I found really hard about losing weight, was that everything was negative ... you couldn't eat this, you couldn't eat that...that was banned, this was banned. No alcohol, no biscuits with tea...ahhhh...it was all just so incredibly negative.

I had so much weight to lose, but it just felt like a horrible endless negative road stretching out ahead of me. So I gave up. I couldn't face the months, years of denying myself.

I think a lot of people give up because of this reason – you just get fed up with punishing yourself constantly with no obvious results or benefits from it. When you've got 50lbs to lose, shifting two or three a week doesn't feel like you're making much of a dent in the problem.

The way things changed for me was when I suddenly started to decide to be really positive about it all. I know this sounds a bit naff, and new age, but let me explain it like this ...

I've always been really bad with money, hopeless at saving (very good at spending), and would never have a very good grip on my finances. I was mortgaged up to my eyeballs, and resented paying it every month for a small house in a very average area. Then one day I went on to Zoopla – the website that tells you how much your house is worth, and I discovered that my house had gone up in value by 12% since I bought it. In that instant I suddenly saw my whole mortgage payments in a much more positive light ... my house was actually worth a decent amount of money ... things weren't that bad. I suddenly became more interested in paying as much of the mortgage off as possible, and became good at saving money rather than spending it, because I wanted to get that mortgage paid off because I suddenly felt more positive and excited about my financial situation.

Exactly the same thing happened with weight loss -- I resented going to the gym, I resented the fact that I wasn't losing much weight, I resented having to cut back foods that I enjoyed ... I just resented everything. Then I went to the gym one time and the woman on reception said "blimey you look great -- you look like you've lost a lot of weight." I'd only lost about seven pounds, but I can't tell you what difference that comment made to me in that moment.

Suddenly I saw the whole thing in a much more positive light. At the gym that day I was determined to run further and exercise harder than I ever have before, and I came home and didn't fancy eating anything unhealthy I wanted to eat things were good for me because I'd enjoyed that moment of positivity. It was exactly the same feeling that I'd had with my house, when I discovered it was worth more than I expected. Positivity is an amazing thing!

Weight-wise, that comment changed everything for me ... suddenly losing weight had gone from a negative to a positive thing. From then on I arrived at the gym feeling good because someone had noticed that I looked better, this meant me wanting to go to the gym more often which led to me losing more weight and toning up further and more good comments, and it all spiralled in a very positive way and allowed me to lose a lot of weight. I've lost 50lbs and I've never felt better.

If I were to give people one reason why I managed to lose the weight it's because I got myself into a positive frame of mind about weight loss ... I started to look at healthy food as being good, and was excited at the fact that I got through a day without eating any rubbish, because it would make me look good in the end, and make me healthier. There is no doubt, for me, that the random comment by a woman whose name I still don't know, made a massive difference, because she hit me with something positive when I felt that everything was very negative. So my advice to you would be to try your hardest to look at your weight loss in a really positive way ... think of all the good things that will come out of it, don't think about the pain of exercising, think about how fabulous you going to look.

Look at the tuna salad you are about to eat, and instead of thinking -- I wish I had a Chinese takeaway -- just think about how much good it is doing you, how much better you are going to feel in the long run, and how amazing you are to be doing this for yourself. Surround yourself with positive people, and read positive things. Watch positive, uplifting videos on You Tube, and the great sports quotes which offer motivational tips. Just read them, read them again and don't allow any negativity to creep in. Keep that positivity up and when you start to lose the weight and start to feel better, you'll end up on the same cycle - feeling positive about weight loss and managing, finally, to shed the unwanted pounds properly and get yourself to a much healthier weight.

Kate's story: Be nice to yourself

Hi, my name is Kate. I'm 67-years-old and I have lost 30lbs. I went from 170lbs to 140lbs. I did it by strict calorie counting. It wasn't easy, but I found it got much easier when I started being nice to myself.

My story:

I'm sure this must look like an odd tip to give you, but by being nice to yourself I mean respect yourself as much as anything. If you are eating too much and have put on weight, you may have given yourself the wrong impression that you're doing this because you're treating yourself to nice food, takeaways and dinner out. The way I lost weight is by learning that I wasn't treating myself nicely by filling myself with food. This was not a nice way to treat myself – it was cruel, heartbreaking and led to me being disappointed, sad and lonely. When I was feeling fat and horrid I didn't want go out and see my friends, I felt ashamed and sad. Is there anyone on earth who would describe putting yourself in this position as being nice to yourself?

No.

It's horrible.

Listen to me – I'm telling you – filling yourself with food is not 'being nice to yourself'. It's not. If you're doing that, you need to stop. Don't beat yourself up, don't have horrible voices in your head telling you how awful you are that you need to eat to feel better. Just stop doing it. Think of it as being nice to yourself, because that's what it is.

My tip is to think about the things you can do today that will make the you of tomorrow much happier. Maybe it's walking a mile a day, maybe it's cutting out sugar, fat, going to Weight Watchers, whatever you want to do to lose the weight – own it, and smile at it. The mindset I adopted was that this was for me... I wasn't punishing myself, I was looking after myself.

I lost weight through calorie counting, and by going to Zumba classes at the gym. I joined a diet group, and when I first started going, I hated the lady who ran it, who would preach at me and all the others there and tell us what we could and couldn't eat. Then I hated the Zumba teacher who shouted at us to jump higher skip higher, put more effort into it.

But then I had a mindset change and I realised that all these people wanted me to be a happier person. They weren't doing it to upset me, or cause me grief. It was only my own head doing that.

So I decided to be nice to myself and to believe everyone else was being nice to me...and it worked. Feeling better and happier genuinely worked.

When I went to Zumba and they told me to work harder, I convinced myself it was because they wanted me to be the best possible version of myself. And when the diet group leader went on and on about vegetable soup I stopped thinking "shut up, leave me alone" and I started thinking – she's giving me this advice because she really cares and knows it really works.

I started realising that the people who were giving me weight watching advice were trying to treat me properly, and the voices in my head telling me to have another cake, and not worry about it, and to dismiss these experts, were not treating me properly. The voices had to change, not my efforts to lose weight.

Obviously, it would have been much easier to stop going to diet club and stop going to Zumba and sit at home eating cakes, but once I'd made that mental transition, that it was important for me to be nice to myself and that being nice to myself involved doing things that were good for my health, the motivation grew and grew and the weight started to fall off.

There were hiccups along the way, of course – an unexpected meal out with friends when I ate too much and drank too much, but I didn't beat myself up – every time my diet and exercise plan went wrong, I just resumed the diet the next day. Don't be afraid of failure, don't beat yourself up when you fail, smile and remember that the most important thing is to treat yourself properly.

Paul's story: I got my self-esteem back.

Hi, my name is Paul. I'm 62-years-old and I have lost 78bs. I went from 248lbs to 170lbs and I did it by getting my self-esteem sorted.

There is no doubt that there is a link between how you feel about yourself and how you treat yourself. If you feel confident, happy and outgoing, then you eat foods that make you feel confident, happy and outgoing. Similarly if you're feeling low and depressed and fed up, you reach for foods that will exacerbate that feeling. If you're in the cycle of feeling rubbish and eating rubbish, you've got to do something to get out of it. You've got to try and eat better and exercise more to make yourself feel better to get yourself into the positive cycle. As we all know (or why would you bought this book?) that's much easier said than done. You have probably tried dieting, as I had, tried exercising, as I had, and couldn't get out of the negative cycle. So, you could try doing what I did - I turned the cycle on its head, and decided to start treating myself better in the hope that that would make me eat better. It worked!

Remember just how much our emotional state impacts upon our physical state. Even the word disease comes from dis-ease... feeling dis at ease with ourselves. Emotional state is really important to your physical state, and that can depend on the environment you are in, the people you're socialising with, the stress you're under, how happy you are, how secure you are and how fulfilled you feel. I felt as if my self-esteem was really low, so I set about doing these six things, and challenging myself in these six areas, which put me in a better frame of mind to focus on getting myself superslim and superfit. And it worked – big time! I've lost over 75lbs.

So, these are the questions I asked myself:

Do I have a low self-esteem?

The easiest way to work this out is to describe yourself in a couple of sentences to an imaginary person in front of you. Do this now before reading any further on. OK. Done that? Then write down the adjectives you used when you described yourself.

This is a sentence that I used: "I'm a fat middle-aged man who is balding, lazy, gets lonely, but is quite nice to his friends."

I didn't realise how low my self-esteem was before I did this test, but experts think that the first words you use to describe yourself are very telling in terms of how you feel about yourself. I know this sounds a bit naff and hippyish, but I made myself look into the mirror every morning and say positive things about myself, reversing the sentences I had used to describe myself.

Horrible head chat

The second thing I made myself do was to talk about myself nicely. You know we all do that thing where we make a simple mistake and in our heads we say "you absolute idiot, what the hell are you doing, can't you do anything right?" Well, I fought very hard to stop it. As soon as I heard myself criticizing myself or putting myself down, I'd tell myself off. Indeed I wrote SHHC on my hand to remind myself to stop the horrible head chat. You can feel it coming on and you can stop it if you try. It doesn't happen at first, but if you keep trying you will stop it and you will feel a whole lot happier and nicer once it goes away.

Accept yourself

You are what you are, and you cannot change how you are in this instant. All you can do is make little changes to improve yourself for the future. But right now there is nothing you can do besides accept who you. In particular, try to accept the vulnerable or not-so-pretty parts of yourself; everyone has these; for example, it is not bad to be anxious or sad sometimes. If you hate walking into a crowded room, don't beat yourself up. Work on conquering the problems, but never think they make you bad or somehow less than other people.

Accept your bad bits as well is your good bits

No one is all good. Don't believe that for a minute. We are all made up of 1 million different bits and pieces – some of the bits are good and some other bits are bad. If you let yourself be defined by the bad bits you'll feel horrible. Think of all the good things you do... the friendships you have, the kindness you show your pets, the way in which you have managed to plant a lovely garden, keep the house clean and tidy. There are lots and lots of good things. We are more than a sum of the bad things, so focus on the good stuff too.

Don't just take criticism

I don't think you should ignore criticism, in fact you should be able to take criticism, but you should always exercise your own judgement when someone criticizes you. Separate criticism out into criticism that is valid, not valid, semi-valid and irrelevant. Make sure you just respond to the valid criticism only, and don't sink into a packet of chips if people criticise you unfairly – tell them.

Treat yourself as if you matter

How on earth are you supposed to eat properly, exercise properly and look after yourself if deep down within your psychology you think you're worthless? Make sure you encourage yourself to do the things you want to do, and give yourself time to be happy and nurtured. It's not your job to runaround making sure everyone else is happy all the time. You matter too!! Whether it's shoveling leftovers into your mouth, rushing around to make sure you're never late for anyone, or dashing to get everything ready for everyone else leaving you only half ready ... whatever it is (mothers be particularly aware - your kids are important but you matter too!!!!), look after yourself. I mean that. You've probably been over-eating for a reason. Take it from me - as someone who went through this and came out the other side - you are worth more than left-overs, second place and scraps!!!! No one in the world is more important than you. You are precious. Look after yourself.

Smile, count your blessings & don't worry.

Being overweight is tough...it affects every part of your life but worrying about it isn't going to help. Infact, worrying about it is going to make everything much harder for you. Stress can paralyse you and thwart all your chances of losing weight.

So – smile, think of three wonderful things in your life, then go for a 10 minute walk.

That's all. You can easily build-up...just do one small thing to get started

Take it slowly, enjoy life, and SMILE.

SECTION FOUR:

WAW! Water and walking

This section is simple, straightforward but vital. There are two things that I really want you to do when you're on your diet campaign – the first is to walk as much as you possibly can, the second is to drink as much water as possible. I'm not saying that you can never have wine and you have to walk everywhere. I'm saying just do as much of it as you possibly can. Try to have a small bottle or glass of water on your desk all the time, and try to make yourself get up and walk around...even for 10 minutes. If you can walk to work instead of driving – great – but even if it's just a walk around the office or to the end of the garden. Do as much as you possibly can.

Water is vital to fill you up and make you feel satisfied, and walking will make you feel better, healthier and as if you are looking after yourself. I promise you: if you do these two things, you WILL feel better and look better.

Water

Some of the readers who have contacted me have spoken about how important water was when they started listening to their bodies and only eating when they were hungry. Often they found they were thirsty rather than hungry. It also filled them up after exercising so they didn't feel the need to eat. A lot of the exercisers spoke about the difficulty of exercising and then being starving afterwards and wanting to eat, thus undoing some of the good work of the exercise. Drinking lots of water helped a great deal with this.

Some of the people I spoke to talked about feeling more alert when they had drunk water, and not getting headaches that they had been getting. Their energy levels lifted and their skin improved. Having improved skin might not necessarily lead directly to weight loss, but as you read through the tips in this book, you'll realise that many successful weight losers state "feeling good" as an important part of what enabled them to shift the weight.

It's important to remember that water makes up almost 70% of our bodies, with some of our internal organs containing even more (the liver is almost all water – some 95%, and remember the liver is responsible for breaking down fatty acids and transporting them to the blood so looking after the liver is important in weight loss. If you don't drink enough water, your liver cannot function properly to metabolise fat and remove toxins from the system).

So from a health perspective it is very important to take a lot of water in. Water also has the job of taking nutrients around the body. If you're cutting back on the food you're eating, you really want the nutrients you take in to be used properly by your body. Water does this, as well as acting as a catalyst for water soluble vitamins.

There is also the odd fact that drinking water helps get rid of water retention. The body retains water when it doesn't get enough of it, so as you start drinking more water your body will let go of the water it has been storing. You notice this in puffy faces and ankles.

The amount of water you should consume every day does vary depending on your height weight and fat loss goals, but as a ballpark figure you should be aiming for a gallon of water a day (so – around eight pints – which sounds a lot, but give it a go and see how many you can manage – any increase is good, and will help). That means a couple of glasses in the morning, a glass before each meal, and a few other glasses scattered through the day.

The other thing about drinking water, is that it stops you from having drinks that are no good for you: fizzy drinks, milky drinks and alcoholic drinks have a lot of sugar and/or fat in them that you can eliminate if you opt for water instead.

This isn't a secret tip or anything, but I pass it on to you because it's a fact that every single person I spoke to who had lost a lot of weight, said they had upped their intake of water considerably.

Walking

Walking is a great way to get light exercise and fresh air. Walking helps you to relax and calm down. Walking is good for your sanity. Go walking – do yourself a favour. Everyone who lost the weight spoke about the value of walking a lot.

Is there any way that you can walk to work, or walk some of the way?

When walking swing your arms faster...if you swing your arms more, you'll find yourself walking more quickly and you'll get your heart rate up.

Just get up and walk around for 5 minutes every hour.

Trey really hard to walk as much as you can. You will be amazed at the difference it makes to your weight.

One of my readers, called Jane, said that you tried everything to lose weight, and it was only when she incorporated exercise that the weight started dropping off. This is her story:

Re-think exercise

Hi, my name is Jane. I'm 25-years-old and I have lost 30lbs. I went from 160lbs to 130lbs. I did it by adding exercise into my daily routine.

My story:

Like lots of women, I never liked exercise. I always thought of it as such a pain – not just the running around bit, but the getting changed in a crowded changing room, then the showering, drying hair, getting changed afterwards.

When I put on weight after my baby was born, I couldn't think of anything worse than taking my huge, fat body into the gym! I was 21, massively overweight, and with a baby to look after. Weight loss was a distant dream.

So, I cut back on unhealthy foods, and some weight started to come off, but I wasn't really committed to it...I'd have some good days, some bad days.

A friend said that by exercising I'd speed up the weight loss, and I'd look better because I'd tone up, making me look as if I'd lost more weight than I actually had. I understood the logic, but – really? It would involve parading my unfit body for all to see. The idea of being sweaty, red-faced and panting with my hair sticking up like a witch, big rolls of fat on my belly and bum shaking with every step ... no thanks.

The thing that made me change my mind about exercise was through rethinking the whole thing. Exercise didn't have to me into going to the gym, it could mean dancing, walking, gentle swimming, a game of gentle tennis ... it didn't have to mean humiliation, it could be fun, and it would help.

So I started walking.

The nice thing about walking your way to fitness is that you can start very gently and build up ... either by going faster or further as you progress. I started to set myself goals ... could I get to the end of the park in 10 minutes. Then could I get to the end of the park and back in 15 minutes. It became a challenge to beat the record I was setting myself. Playing music while I did it meant it was actually quite an uplifting experience, and it made me feel better getting more fresh air and being out and about more than I had been.

I'd always justified to myself that I wouldn't exercise because it was so painful, and also because everything I read said that it was much easier to lose weight through diet than through exercise. Even when I looked at all the research that had been done ... googling how much weight you could expect to lose with exercise, all the research was showing there was hardly any weight loss with exercise alone.

But what I found when I did it was that there were lots of benefits – it's motivating, because when you exercise as well as diet, you see changes quicker because you tone up, so it inspires you to lose more weight.

Also, remember that exercise, even if it doesn't result in direct weight loss, has a hugely beneficial impact on the body and a massive psychological impact. If I'd made the effort to get up in the morning and walk for half an hour before work, the last thing I wanted to do was eat a fatty breakfast and undo all the good when I got back.

In terms of the physical impact of exercise, most of the effects are well known...good for your heart, your bones, your muscles and your lungs. I discovered that there's also an added benefit for people like me who have yo-yo dieted so much that their metabolism is thrown completely out of sync. My doctor said that exercise can help fix a metabolism that is wrecked by yo-yo dieting. If you don't exercise your metabolism slows down, if you start moving again it will start to change and start to become better. If you've ever been obese, your metabolism will have suffered. One of the best things you can do to get your metabolism is back on track as possible is to start moving ... any gentle exercise at all will really help. It did for me.

A note from Bernie: 70% of the people who contacted me with their weight loss tips for this book said that they had done some form of physical activity as part of their weight-loss campaign. Even if it was just going for a gentle stroll a couple of times a week ... people found it helped to include activity of some sort into their lives.

Bus drivers

OK, I'm going to tell you a story now, so relax, put your feet up and listen very carefully. I'm going to take you back to 1949 when an interesting study was done by Jerry Morris, a professor of social medicine.

Morris noticed that bus drivers, as a group, had way more heart-attacks than other groups of workers. They were also fatter than many other groups of workers. He understood the link between heart disease and obesity, but why bus drivers? What was going on?

He wanted to compare the drivers with people in similar professions, who has similar stresses and similar lifestyles, so he decided to compare London bus drivers and London bus conductors. The drivers and conductors were from similar social backgrounds; however, there was a marked difference in the rates of disease between the two groups.

Morris conducted an analysis which showed that, compared to drivers, conductors were half as likely to die from a heart attack. He also spent many hours riding buses, building a profile of the daily routines of drivers and conductors. His explanation for the bus drivers' ailing bodies was that in a working day, while drivers were typically sedentary, conductors walked around all day.

The difference between conductors and drivers was that conductors walked, and because of that – it seemed – they were half as likely to die. Now, obviously, there could have been other factors at play – one could argue that driving a bus is more stressful a job, but there was no doubt to researchers that the walking they were doing was saving their lives.

This was really one of the first times doctors began to appreciate the link between early death and an inactive, sedentary life or, conversely, the protective effects of physical activity. Being overweight or obese wasn't taken much into account back then as many of the drivers were of normal weight. Now, over 60 years later, the link between a sedentary life and early death has been reconfirmed in dozens of studies worldwide.

So – please – walk whenever you can. Try and squeeze in a walk whenever you can. It's really important.

Bernice Bloom

SECTION FIVE:
Making it a habit

All these things are great to do, they are simple and they really don't take long at all, but you have to do them regularly to make a difference. We're all familiar with the way things work - you get into a routine and start developing healthy ways, the weight starts to come off, then you have a bad night and it all collapses, you eat badly, your head goes and suddenly all the weight goes back on, leaving you feeling hopeless as well as overweight.

You can only create new habits by changing your attitude to food and not using it as a crutch. While you're relying on food to get you through tough times, your ability to succeed is limited by events out of your control. One day something difficult happens to make you feel bad and you're at the chocolate biscuits.

You can lose weight, and you can feel really great about yourself, but only if you let yourself believe that it's JUST FOOD, and will not help if your marriage breaks up, your cleaner runs off with the family silver or you lose your job. Food can't help with those things.

You need to create new habits...this is how some readers did it:

Sarah's story: I broke my bad habits & created new ones

Hi, my name is Sarah, I'm 68-years-old and I have lost 50lbs. I went from 196lbs to 146lbs. I did it by sensible eating, and I think the reason I was able to lose weight when so many other people fail, is because I changed my behaviour around food by breaking my lifetime habits.

My story:

I'm so glad I've been asked to share my weight loss tips with you because I have lost 50lbs and I did it by breaking all my bad habits. I think the key to losing weight is to understand what your habits are ... what you do regularly has made you the weight you are. If you don't like that weight - break those habits.

For example, I found myself drinking loads of cups of tea at work, and every time I went to the kettle to make a cup of tea there'd be biscuits there. I'd have a biscuit while the kettle was boiling, make a cup of tea and take it back to my desk with another biscuit. I did that every time. That's around 200 calories every time I made a cup of tea. It was definitely a habit. I wasn't having a biscuit because I was hungry, but because they were there, and it was a nice thing to do while the kettle was boiling.

What I learnt when I started to think about my habit of getting up to have cups of tea all the time was that half the reason I was standing up from my desk was because I felt I needed a break, and to talk to people. It was the same at lunchtime, rather than taking healthy lunch from home, I'd always go to the cafe over the road, because that way I'd meet people and talk to them and get some fresh air. My job is very solitary – I'm a researcher in a library.

So what I decided to do was to accept that what I wanted was interaction with people, and give myself a short break every couple of hours to wander out, get some fresh air and talk to other researchers, then come back to my desk. I didn't need tea and I didn't need the biscuits and I didn't need the calorific sandwiches at lunch time. That was all just habit. Habits can be broken as soon as you identify them.

Do you have a habit of having a glass of wine every night after work? Do you convince yourself that now the bottle's open you might as well have another one? I certainly used to. It's all just habit and it's hundreds and hundreds and thousands of calories you're taking in, just because of bad habits.

It's not the body or your metabolism that's making you overweight or obese – it's your brain. That's really clear to me now, after losing weight that I had been trying to lose for half my life.

It's poor decisions that make you gain weight. Good decisions will allow you to lose it. If you're overweight, you might have been making bad decisions for a while, and the problem is that over time, the poor decisions lead to <u>significant changes</u> in how the brain behaves. Years of any kind of behavior pattern creates habits that take some breaking. The good news is that the brain can "fix" itself once new habits are formed.

You need to rewire your brain. The way to do this is to work out what bad habits you have around food...biscuits with tea, a glass of wine with dinner, extras, pudding, eating crisps. Keep a note of what you're eating during a week and spot patterns. Try and identify just two habits to change and change them.

Work out why you're always eating a chocolate bar on the train on the way home. Is it because you're hungry? If so, have something healthier, if it's not because you're hungry – why? Tiredness, boredom, or just buying one out of habit. You need to understand yourself if you're going to lose weight – work out why you're sabotaging yourself. Once you know why you're always doing something, you can set about trying to change it...make new healthy habits and finally shift that weight.

Philippa's story: I became accountable

Hi, my name is Philippa. I'm 53-years-old and I have lost 44lbs. I went from 210lbs to 166lbs. I did it by making myself accountable. I decided to take weight loss seriously...treated it like a business.

My story:

My tip might sound a bit odd at first – be accountable. To whom? It's only you responsible for your weight. But the gist of my tip for you, as someone who's lost a hell of a lot of weight, and kept it off (for two years now) is to be accountable to yourself. Be organised, plan properly, treat the process like an important business campaign because in many ways it's much more important than that...this is your God damned health we're talking about here...take it seriously!

So, I decided to become accountable .... I decided to weigh myself every Monday at the same time, and keep my weight loss results on a chart next to my desk. Then I made sure I kept a food diary, listing everything I had eaten or drunk that day. I know you read a lot of diet instructions which say that you should keep a food diary, and I'd always dismissed it before, I would definitely, definitely advise doing it because it does help you see what you're eating, and where you could make little cutbacks to help lose weight.

If you make yourself accountable, and keep proper records of everything, it's really motivating when you do well. Also, when you don't do well, you can see exactly where the problems are rising (maybe in that week where you drank too much wine you didn't lose weight, so it reminds you to cut back on the booze). If you haven't kept a record of everything, you don't know how you're doing, and it's very hard to improve.

I know some people aren't naturally planners, or organisers, but even if you're not, if you can bear it you will find you get much better results if you plan carefully, monitor carefully, and record all your results. That's certainly what I found, and if you look at companies like Weight Watchers and the Cambridge diet and all those other formal diets, one of the main things they do is weigh you and give you feedback on your weight and measurements all the time. Even if you do a weight loss program in a gym, they weigh you and measure you at the beginning and give your updates as to how your plan is going. They do this because they know that if you get feedback it helps motivate you. If you're doing it yourself, like I was, you need to provide your own motivation, so you need to get yourself organised and make yourself accountable.

These are the ways I suggest you do it ... this is certainly the way I lost weight:

- Keep a food diary of everything you eat, be as honest as you possibly can, and update it regularly. No one will see this but you, but it does help you realise how you're making slipups along the way, or even to give you something to congratulate yourself on when you have a particularly good day.

- Chart your measurements and weight as the weight starts to come off. Either weigh yourself once a week or once every two weeks - it's up to you, but make sure you keep a record of what's going on.

- Get organised at home. I've found with my diet that the times I wasn't able to keep to it was when I hadn't organised myself properly. I think you have to plan your meals in advance so you know what to buy, so you've always got good food in the house. There's nothing more likely to make you eat badly than a situation where the only food in your house is pizza and crisps. Make sure this doesn't happen by being organised and planning meals in advance.

- Plan to do some exercise ... it's very easy not to do any because you're too busy. I think you have to prioritize it. You never don't eat because you're too busy, you do the things are important. I've found it really worked for me when I prioritized exercise. When I say exercise, sometimes this was going for a swim after work, other times it was just getting off the bus earlier and walking, or walking up the stairs ... just making sure I planned something into the day that counted as exercise.

· Reward yourself. The point of being accountable is that you can praise yourself as well as criticise yourself!

· Be clear about the times you allow yourself to eat. Before I went on my diet I found myself eating quite a lot late at night. I'd come back from work by about six, sort out the kids, get changed into something comfortable pour myself a glass of wine and relax then I was at my most dangerous ... crisps and dips, another glass of wine, cheese sandwich ... Now I have a rule that I must not eat after 6.30 PM unless I'm going out to dinner. So, I come back from work, prepare healthy meal for myself and my kids straight away, then I don't eat again that evening. It's really worked for me, and if I get hungry, I just drink loads and loads of water. Sparkling water is particularly filling.

Some other tips from my readers:

Mike's story: I learnt from McDonalds.

Hi, my name is Mike. I'm 19-years-old and I have lost 50lbs. I went from 270lbs to 220lbs and I did it by realizing what fast food restaurants did to make you eat a lot, and I did the opposite. I'm fairly sure that my diet tip will be the most ridiculous one in this research... it's all about fooling yourself into eating less, eating less frequently, and eating more healthily by taking advice from McDonald's, Burger King, Wimpey, Wendy's and all other fast food outlets.

My story:

I was a junk food addict...eating fast food all the time. I was aware that I'd go into McDonalds and have a burger and fries and immediately want another one, but I thought that was just me being greedy. Then I saw an interesting article about how fast food outlets encourage you to spend more money. They obviously do this by trying to get you to eat more, and eat faster. It struck me that if I tried to do the opposite of what fast food restaurants do, then I would be encouraging myself to eat less and eat more slowly.

So... here are the lessons from McDonald's that can help you lose weight:

1.) In McDonald's they don't have plates -- they put your food onto trays. The reason they do this is to make the food look quite small on the tray, so you don't feel as if you're eating very much. This encourages you to feel as if you can eat much more. So, the first thing I did was serve my food on the smallest plates I had in the house. I'd just give myself a portion that could fit onto a small plates, and if I was still hungry I'd have a little bit more. Apparently this genuinely does work to make you eat less, because when a plate is full it sends messages to your brain that there's a lot of it, so your brain sends a message out that you are full much sooner than it would.

2.) In McDonald's they put food flat onto the tray, this is because when food is piled up it makes you feel as if you're eating more, so when you serve yourself at home put your food into a tall pile and it makes it look as if you've got a lot more of it (I know this sounds odd, but it's true!)

3.)   McDonald's restaurants are deliberately unatmospheric; they don't want you to linger in there when you're not eating. You are not encouraged to stay for a coffee afterwards. The music they play is tinny, not conducive to sitting around for a long time while you eat. This is what makes you eat more quickly. So I started making an effort to lay the table properly, sit down with a nice atmosphere, and relish my food at home, instead of rushing it. I certainly think that if you take more time with your food, you feel yourself getting full-up more quickly, and don't reach for seconds.

4.)   In McDonald's the lights are very bright, this is another way of making you eat faster. That's why lovely, expensive restaurants have candlelight.

5.)   The colours ... the colours red and yellow are designed to make you want to eat, that's why McDonald's uses them. Apparently, blue is the colour that least makes you want to eat. So, next time you go to buy any new crockery, go for small plates and plates that are either blue, or white with a blue pattern (again -- the colours that you would associate with a smart restaurant).

I know this may sound like a silly tip, but I'm being honest. Iit was when I stopped rushing my food, ate slowly, and didn't behave like a teenager in a

McDonald's restaurant, that I started to really move the weight. I've actually lost 50lbs, so I desperately needed to lose weight. It was the little tricks that helped me. I wish you lots and lots of luck in your efforts to lose weight. Be kind to yourself, treat yourself nicely, and whatever you do don't behave like a starving teenager in a McDonald's restaurant.

Jen's story: Tapping

Hi, my name is Jen. I'm 53-years-old and I have lost 40lbs. I went from 180lbs to 140lbs and I did it by learning the art of tapping. I find it calms me down, gives me breathing space and has stopped my frenetic eating.

My story:

OK, before we start, I should tell you that this is nothing to do with tap dancing. When I told my husband that I was going to try tapping to lose weight, he said straight away "well don't do it in here, we have wooden floors, the guys in the apartment downstairs will be horrified." But it's nothing to do with dance. Tapping is a way of relaxing yourself, getting control of yourself, and getting rid of urges and this all happens by tapping yourself with your fingers.

I'm well aware of how ridiculous this all sounds, but by tapping certain parts of your face arms and shoulders that have been identified as linked to urges, you do manage to get control over yourself, and stop eating so much. At least I did.

My tip is to try tapping – what have you got to lose? It definitely, definitely worked for me. I'm 53 now, and when I was 48 I'd almost given up hope of ever losing weight. I saw tapping mentioned in a newspaper article, and gave it a go. I bought a book, but I don't think you even need to do that, you just need to know where to tap, and when to do it, and if you're anything like me it will make all the difference in the world. I don't know how or why – I don't understand any of the science behind it (though apparently there's lots of science behind it), all I know is that the theory is that it helps bridge the gap between your body and your mind, allowing you to do a small physical movement that sends a strong signal to the brain.

So, below I've listed exactly what I did to lose weight through tapping. It's just a few stages, but it is worth going through these stages properly for you to have the maximum benefit.

Stage One

The hardest thing about losing weight through tapping is that you have to work out what is making you eat in the first place. So you will have to spend a bit of time thinking about yourself, and what is making you behave the way you are. If you always have something to eat after a row with your kids, a row with the boss, or a difficult commute into work – these are the things that you are going to be tapping to get rid of. You can tap directly to get rid of your desire to eat all the time, or your anger that you've put on so much weight, but I personally started doing this, then the more I read about it, realise that the more specific the thing you are tapping for, the greater the results.

I realised that I was reaching out for food when I got off the train after my really stressful commute to work every morning. By tapping away the stress I felt, I stopped myself eating the half a packet of biscuits, crisps and cakes that I had once consumed.

This worked for me, because I had established before starting tapping that it was my stressful commute that was causing me the most emotional pressure, and most likely lead me to emotional eating. I recommend that you do this first before starting the tapping.

Stage Two

Next, you need to work out how much stress you're feeling in certain circumstances – do this simply by thinking about yourself in a situation...dealing with your boss, when the baby is crying, when you're trying to sort out your finances ... whatever it is, write a score down for how angry, cross or upset it makes you feel. If you don't feel anything at all about that particular scenario, give it a zero. This bit is all about gut instinct, so don't think about it for too long -- just write down whatever you're feeling, and give it a score.

Stage Three

You need to create a statement which encompasses how you are feeling (ie: stressed about the commute), but in the statement you say that you won't let the feeling control you.

So, my statement was: 'I acknowledge that I feel stressed and angry when I drive into work, I accept how I feel and I am OK.'

The one I did specifically mentioning weight loss was: "Even though I am angry that I have put on three stone, I accept who I am, and I'm OK.'

One friend I spoke to said she didn't feel 'angry' at putting on weight, but very, very upset, so she changed the word 'angry' for 'upset' – you need to get this word right, because it's that emotion that we're trying to banish.

Stage four

This is where you get tapping:

There are 10 stages – do each of these while saying your statement three times in each phase.

1.   Tap with two fingers from one hand on the fleshy part of the hand below the little finger on the other hand, while saying your statement three times.

2.   Tap inside the eyebrow, while saying your statement three times.

3.   Tap the outer edge of the eye, while saying your statement three times.

4.   Tap under your eye, at the lower edge of the eye socket, while saying your statement three times.

5.   Tap under your nose, while saying your statement three times.

6.   Tap under your chin, while saying your statement three times.

7.   Tap your collarbone, while saying your statement three times.

8.   Tap your armpit, while saying your statement three times.

9.   Tap the top of your head, while saying your statement three times.

Now ask yourself whether you feel better about the issues that led you to over eat. Rate yourself again and see whether your number has dropped...if it has – brilliant! Repeat that every day. Eventually you can move to a more positive statement: 'I'm happy that I no longer eat all the time and feel I have control over myself'.

I know this might not work for everyone, and I know how daft it sounds, but it worked brilliantly for me.

CONCLUSION

So...there you have it. Some tips from me and from my readers who have got in touch. If you want to share any tips with me, any funny stories or observations, please do, and we'll add them onto the website and include them in new editions of this book.

To end this book, I'd just like to repeat something that I wrote at the beginning:

If you are overweight it's not because you're a bad person, you didn't kill anyone, you didn't steal anything, or hit anyone, or do anything criminal. You just ate too much because you felt low, or got into a habit of eating while bored. That's not a crime. Most importantly, it can be changed.

If you eat a bag of chips tonight or eight packet of biscuits, the world won't end, just shrug it off, wake up tomorrow and try to go for a 10 minute walk and have a glass of water. No one ever lost weight by beating themselves up and feeling bad.

For any information about my novels, or to join the mailing list, please see the website: www.bernicebloom.com. There is a weight loss community on there, featuring a weight loss and nutrition news section that is updated every day to bring you the latest news from all around the world.

Bernie x

Printed in Great Britain
by Amazon

80286957R00079